I0446550

HYPNO THERAPY SIMPLIFIED

Unlock Your Potential And Transform Your Life, A Comprehensive Guide To The Core Techniques, Healing, Targeted Applications, And Key Principle

DR. LILIAN AUDREY

Disclaimer:

The data in this book, "HypnoTherapy Simplified," is solely meant to be informative and instructional.

This book is not intended to replace expert medical advice, diagnosis, or care. No medical, health, or other professional services are offered by the author, publisher, or any affiliated parties

Individual outcomes may differ in the practice of these therapies, which entail a variety of approaches and methodologies.

A one-on-one session with a trained or certified healthcare professional is still preferable. It is best to consult a trained healthcare provider before making any decisions regarding your health.

The author of this book is not affiliated with any specific website, product, or organization related to any of these therapies.

All reasonable measures have been taken by the author and publisher to guarantee the authenticity and dependability of the material contained in this book.

Contents

About the book

Understanding Hypnosis

Clarifies what hypnosis is, how it functions, and busts myths and misconceptions about this healing modality.

The function of the hypnotherapist, the therapeutic process, induction methods, and ways to sustain and deepen a hypnotic state are all covered

The Practice of Hypnotherapy.

Applications of Hypnotherapy

delves into the various uses of hypnosis, such as managing pain, reducing stress and anxiety, overcoming phobias, losing weight and adopting a healthy diet, quitting smoking, enhancing self-esteem, controlling addictions, and improving performance and creativity.

Hypnotherapy for Mental Health

Covers the application of hypnosis in the treatment of mental health issues, including depression, PTSD, trauma, grieving, and loss; it also covers building connections and resilience.

Specialized Hypnosis Techniques

Explores specialized uses such as parts therapy, age regression, previous life regression, and hypnosis for kids and teenagers.

The ethical components of hypnotherapy,

such as informed consent, secrecy, and privacy,: Ethical Considerations

Self-Hypnosis and Self-Care

will enable readers to learn how to hypnotize themselves, write scripts for self-hypnosis, and utilize hypnosis as a tool for self-improvement.

Research and Future Directions

looks at the future of this field, scientific research on hypnosis, and an examination of the therapeutic efficacy.

To deepen their awareness of hypnotherapy and its therapeutic potential, readers will also discover a wealth of useful materials and references.

This book offers a thorough and educational introduction to the field of hypnotherapy, catering to readers who may be interested in learning more about the various applications, the science underlying hypnosis, or ethical issues surrounding self-hypnosis.

CHAPTER ONE

Hypnotherapy: What Is It?

Similar to hypnosis, hypnotherapy is a complementary therapy that has become well-known for its ability to treat a variety of mental and physical problems.

The main goals of hypnotherapy are to induce a heightened state of awareness, or hypnosis, by concentrated attention and guided relaxation.

People in this changed state are more receptive to recommendations and therapeutic interventions meant to address a range of issues, from pain management and smoking cessation to anxiety and phobias.

The Background Of Hypnosis

Historical accounts of trance-like states and hypnotic procedures go back thousands of years, which is where the origins of hypnotherapy can be found.

In their healing rituals and spiritual practices, people from many nations and communities have used hypnosis or trance states, from the Indigenous peoples of the Americas to ancient Egypt.

But it wasn't until the 18th and 19th centuries that hypnosis received widespread recognition in the West, largely as a result of the contributions of individuals like Franz Mesmer and James Braid.

Hypnosis was made possible by the introduction of the theory of "animal magnetism" by the Austrian physician Franz Mesmer in the late 1700s.

The 19th-century Scottish surgeon James Braid is credited with creating the term "hypnosis" and expanding our knowledge of this altered state of awareness.

Hypnotherapy made strides in the 20th century and was incorporated into several therapeutic modalities, including cognitive-behavioral therapy and psychoanalysis.

It is increasingly acknowledged as a valid and efficient therapy approach for treating a variety of emotional and psychological issues.

Hypnosis's Scientific Basis

Extensive research and inquiry have been conducted to understand the science behind hypnosis.

The functioning of hypnosis has been clarified by modern neuroscience and psychology, even though the precise mechanisms at work are still unknown.

Essentially, it seems that hypnosis activates certain brain areas linked to suggestibility, focused attention, and altered perception.

Research employing brain imaging methods, such as functional magnetic resonance imaging (fMRI), has demonstrated that the brain's default mode network, which is in charge of indulging in self-referential ideas and daydreaming, becomes less active during hypnosis. Concurrently, there is increased activity in the areas related to perception, memory, and executive function.

In hypnotherapy, the power of suggestion is a key component. Hypnosis makes people more responsive to therapeutic recommendations, which enables a range of difficulties to be addressed, from habit modification to pain management and anxiety reduction.

With their techniques and applications, hypnotherapy and hypnosis are complementary holistic approaches to well-being.

While hypnotherapy addresses psychological and emotional issues by using altered states of consciousness, hypnosis concentrates on the physical manipulation of soft tissues to induce relaxation and ease physical discomfort.

Each adds to the larger field of holistic health and wellness uniquely.

Revealing The Healing Potential Of Hypnosis

As a well-known and successful method of encouraging relaxation, reducing stress, and enhancing physical well-being, hypnotherapy has gained popularity.

The idea of honor as a therapeutic technique has developed over the ages, meeting the demands of both physical and mental health, with roots in ancient cultures. We will examine the many facets and advantages of hypnotherapy as we delve into this intriguing field in this post.

The Hypnotic State: A Transcending Experience For The Mind

Since the purpose of both therapies is to promote relaxation and well-being, it's crucial to comprehend the concept of hypnosis before delving into the world of hypnotherapy.

A condition of intense concentration and increased suggestibility, hypnosis is frequently accompanied by profound relaxation.

A person in hypnosis is not under the hypnotist's control, despite how this is frequently portrayed in popular culture; rather, they are in a condition of increased openness to suggestions.

How Hyno Operates: Revealing The Touch Art

The major medium used in hypnotherapy is the therapeutic value of human touch. Skilled hypnotists utilize a range of methods, including friction, petrissage, and effleurage, to work with the body's soft tissues.

These methods increase blood flow, ease tense muscles, and bring about a deep state of relaxation.

In addition to relieving physical suffering, the therapist's deft use of pressure, strokes, and kneading movements has a tremendous effect on mental health.

The way hypnotherapy functions is by inducing the body's healing mechanisms.

The body gets more adept at eliminating waste and supplying vital nutrients to cells when circulation and lymphatic drainage are enhanced.

This procedure improves general physical well-being, decreases inflammation, and speeds up tissue repair.

Furthermore, Hyno's art transcends the tangible. A professional therapist's soothing and consoling touch can induce profound relaxation, reducing stress and promoting mental peace.

The body and mind can repair, revitalize, and heal when they are in this relaxed state.

Myths & False Beliefs Regarding Hypnotherapy

Hypnotherapy, like hypnosis, is not without its myths and misconceptions. A prevalent misperception is that hypnotherapy is an extravagance only to the wealthy.

In actuality, it provides observable health advantages, making it useful and accessible to a diverse group of people.

A further misconception is that hypnosis is exclusive to people with physical illnesses or wounds.

Although it is a useful technique for treating musculoskeletal problems, those who want to relax, de-stress, and improve their mental health can also benefit from it.

Moreover, it is untrue to say that hypnotherapy is essentially a pampering procedure.

It is certainly a pleasant experience, but it goes beyond just coziness. A competent therapist's healing touch has the power to raise general health, strengthen emotional well-being, and increase quality of life.

Utilizing the natural healing properties of human touch, hypnosis is a flexible and effective therapeutic approach.

It is comparable to hypnosis in that it can induce deep relaxation in people, which opens the door to both mental and physical health.

People can discover the many advantages of hypnotherapy by dispelling misconceptions and realizing its purpose, which makes it a crucial part of a holistic approach to health and well-being.

Hyno As Therapy: Uncovering Touch's Healing Potential

Hypnotherapy is an all-encompassing therapeutic method that uses the natural power of touch.

This age-old method has shown to be a remarkably powerful therapeutic tool that cuts across both time and cultural boundaries.

Hypnotherapists are sought after by that seeking pain treatment, relaxation, and improved well-being because they are skilled in navigating the intricate terrain of human emotions, physiology, and senses.

In this examination of hypnotherapy, we get into the complex idea of touch as a powerful tool for healing and talk about the varied functions that hypnotherapists play in the therapeutic process.

CHAPTER TWO

Hypnotherapy Practice: Unlocking The Potential Of The Mind

Hypnotherapy is a therapeutic modality that works by accessing the subconscious to bring about significant transformations and healing.

It is directed by the skillful hands and perceptive brains of hypnotists, who recognize that the human mind may be a maze-like place.

Beyond merely putting patients into a trance, hypnotherapy is a purposeful trip into the subconscious, where significant changes take place.

The Hypnotherapist's Role: Getting Through The Subconscious

A competent hypnotherapist is a kind guide through the maze-like passageways of the subconscious.

They create secure, caring spaces that encourage openness, trust, and discovery; they are the designers of therapeutic landscapes.

They have an acute sense of intuition and can discern the particular requirements of each client, customizing their strategy to fit that person's journey.

The hypnotherapist has a responsibility to act with compassion, comprehension, and deep regard for the inner workings of the human mind.

The Healing Process: Dividing Into Inner Truths

The therapeutic procedure in the field of hypnotherapy is a complex dance between the therapist and the patient.

It's a nuanced interaction between suggestions, language, and mental flexibility. Hypnotherapists work to identify the underlying causes of medical illnesses, undesired behaviors, and emotional discomfort while fostering a safe and encouraging environment.

To uncover and resolve deeply ingrained issues, the client and therapist collaborate throughout the therapy process.

Induction Methodologies: Handling The Subconscious Portal

The keys that open the door to the subconscious mind are induction procedures. Hypnotherapists promote heightened receptivity in their clients through relaxation, visualization, and concentrated concentration.

These methods can be tailored to each client's specific requirements and tastes, making them as varied as the clients themselves.

Being able to gently lead a client into a deep state of relaxation and inner attention is the art of induction.

CHAPTER THREE

Deepening And Preserving Hypnosis: Continuing The Healing Process

For a session to be successful, deepening and maintaining hypnosis is essential after the subconscious door has been established.

To maintain the client in the therapeutic trance, hypnotherapists employ a range of techniques, such as creative metaphors, progressive relaxation, and calming verbal cues.

Initiating transformative change, identifying underlying causes, and exploring inner landscapes are all made possible by this elevated state of consciousness.

The tremendous healing powers of the mind and the power of touch are combined in the fields of hypnotherapy and hypnotherapy.

Although hypnotherapists and hypnotherapists work in distinct fields, they are always committed to promoting their customers' well-being.

Touch and the subconscious are the guiding lights of the healing path, which is a deeply interrelated one, as both techniques show great regard for the subtle balance between the body and mind.

Hypnotherapy: An All-Inclusive Method Of Recovery

The time-tested method of hypnotherapy has gained popularity as a potent therapeutic approach with uses in many different areas of health and well-being. Because of its adaptability, it can be used to treat a wide range of medical and psychological conditions, providing pain relief, reducing stress, and releasing latent potential.

This article examines the many uses of hypnotherapy and highlights how it can improve quality of life and well-being in general.

Habitat Management: Alleviation By Touch

Pain management is one of the most well-known uses of hypnotherapy. A hypnotherapist's expert hands can do wonders for easing and eliminating a variety of pain issues, such as chronic pain syndromes, joint stiffness, and muscular soreness. Hyno helps release endorphins, relax stiff muscles, and increase blood circulation through focused techniques and gentle manipulation, all of which contribute to much-needed discomfort relief.

Reduction Of Stress And Anxiety: A Calm Approach

Stress and worry have become commonplace in today's fast-paced environment. Hypnotherapy provides a peaceful haven where people can relax and let go of the stress that accumulates throughout the day. A hypnotherapy session's relaxing atmosphere and the power of touch can significantly lower stress hormones, encourage relaxation, and lessen anxiety.

Overcoming Fears And Phobias: A Road To Bravery

Hypnotherapy, with its calming effects, might provide a special path to recovery for people struggling with phobias and fears.

Through fostering a feeling of security and calm, Hyno can assist people in facing their fears and eventually developing the bravery to do so.

This therapy strategy offers a nurturing environment for human development and change.

Healthy Eating And Weight Loss: A Holistic Approach

Hypnosis therapy might be an unanticipated ally in the pursuit of healthy living.

It's not a weight-loss method per se, but it does help control weight by lowering stress-related overeating and encouraging awareness.

Hypnosis treatments can help people relax and feel more connected to their bodies, which can facilitate the adoption of healthy eating habits.

Quitting Smoking: Overcoming Addiction

Hypnotherapy can be extremely helpful when trying to quit smoking. This treatment modality tackles the physiological and psychological dimensions of addiction by mitigating withdrawal symptoms, lowering cravings, and offering emotional reinforcement.

The likelihood of successfully stopping smoking can be greatly increased by using this all-encompassing strategy.

Slumber Enhancement: Acquiring Calm During The Night

Hypnotherapy presents a promising solution for individuals suffering from insomnia and sleep difficulties, promising peaceful nights. Hyno's calming effects can aid in controlling sleep cycles and encouraging restful, deep sleep. People can sleep better and be in better health overall by reducing stress and worry.

CHAPTER FOUR

Inner Strength: Increasing Self-Confidence And Self-Esteem

A strong sense of self-acceptance and self-worth is fostered via hypnotherapy. People might improve their confidence and self-image by reestablishing a connection with their bodies through the compassionate touch of a therapist.

The impact of this increased confidence on both personal and professional achievement can be profound.

Overcoming Addictions: A Route To Rehab

Although the fight against addiction might be difficult, hypnosis can be a useful aid in the healing process. Hypno therapy aids in the path to sobriety and a better, addiction-free life by lessening cravings, relieving withdrawal symptoms, and offering emotional support.

Improving Originality And Output: Unlocking Potential

In the fields of performance and creativity, hypnosis acts as a spark to release latent potential.

In the arts, sports, or professional pursuits, it enables people to reach their full potential by lowering stress, improving focus, and fostering a sense of well-being.

Hypnosis is a gentle and adaptable therapy that can be applied to a variety of human experiences.

It provides a comprehensive approach to healing, ranging from reducing physical pain to improving mental health.

Its soft-touch has the power to change lives by encouraging vitality, personal development, and relaxation.

Psychological Hypnotherapy

Hypnotherapy is a special and adaptable kind of mental health care that provides a comprehensive and non-invasive way to deal with a variety of psychological problems.

It makes use of the subconscious mind's ability to assist people in overcoming obstacles, create coping mechanisms, and improve their mental health.

Here, we look at how hypnosis can be used to treat depression, manage trauma and PTSD, deal with loss and sorrow, develop resilience, and enhance relationships.

Weight Loss Treatment

Millions of individuals worldwide are impacted by the complicated and widespread mental health illness known as depression.

Depression treatment can benefit greatly from the use of hypnotherapy.

Hypnotherapy works by exploring the subconscious to find and reframe negative thought patterns, increase self-worth, and facilitate relaxation.

Through improved symptom management, this approach can provide patients hope and relief as they work toward recovery.

Treating Trauma And PTSD

Living with Post-Traumatic Stress Disorder (PTSD) and other illnesses associated with trauma can be extremely difficult. Hypnotherapy provides a secure and powerful method for dealing with these problems.

A professional hypnotherapist can help people process traumatic experiences, lessen the emotional baggage associated with them, and create healthy coping skills by putting them in a condition of increased suggestibility.

Overcoming Loss And Grief

Loss and grief can be crippling, impacting not just our mental health but also our physical health.

By assisting people in exploring their emotions, coming to terms with their losses, and navigating the different stages of grief, hypnotherapy can offer comfort and support during these trying times.

People can discover inner power, get a greater understanding of their emotions, and gradually reclaim a feeling of balance in their lives through hypnosis.

Creating Hardiness

The capacity to overcome hardship is known as resilience, and it is an essential element of mental wellness.

By influencing the subconscious mind to create coping mechanisms, lower anxiety, and inculcate positive attitudes, hypnotherapy can help develop resilience.

This strategy ultimately promotes mental resilience by empowering people to meet life's obstacles with increased strength and self-assurance.

Strengthening Bonds

Good connections might be difficult, but they are necessary for our well-being. Hypnotherapy can help people understand and change their thought patterns, emotional reactions, and communication styles, which can help with relationship problems. Consequently, this can result in more contented and peaceful relationships with family members and friends.

To sum up, hypnotherapy is an effective and comprehensive strategy for enhancing mental wellness.

Through the management of depression, PTSD, trauma, grief, and loss, the development of resilience, and the improvement of relationships, hypnotherapy offers a flexible toolkit to help people manage the intricacies of their inner lives and promote happier, healthier lives.

 To make sure that this therapy is customized to one's unique requirements and problems, it is imperative to speak with a licensed and competent hypnotherapist.

CHAPTER FIVE

Techniques Of Specialized Hypnotherapy

Hypnotherapy is an adaptable method of self-improvement and healing that uses many different specialized approaches.

These methods make use of the subconscious mind's capacity to handle a range of problems and encourage constructive transformation.

Some of the specialist hypnotherapy techniques that will be covered in this talk are Parts Therapy, Age Regression, Past Life Regression, and Hypnotherapy for Children and Adolescents.

Regression To Past Lives

An interesting and contentious area of hypnosis is Past Life Regression. By putting people into a hypnotic state, this approach allows them to access and investigate memories or experiences from what they perceive to be their former lives.

The fundamental principle is based on the notions of reincarnation and the influence of past events or traumas on one's present existence.

Regression to a prior life is a therapeutic technique for identifying and releasing unsolved problems, phobias, or fears thought to be inherited from previous lifetimes.

It has grown in popularity as a way to treat ingrained emotional and psychological issues, while not having any scientific backing.

Regression In Age

Hypnotherapy called "Age Regression" transports patients back in time to their early years, such as childhood or infancy.

Regression is made possible by profound relaxation and targeted suggestion, which gives people the opportunity to relive traumatic experiences or prior events in a secure setting.

Age regression is a useful technique for treating unresolved childhood traumas, unresolved behavioral patterns, or disorders that persist into adulthood.

Reliving these early events can help people develop and heal, let go of emotional baggage, and obtain new perspectives.

Parts Counseling

The hypnotherapeutic technique known as Parts Therapy, or Ego State Therapy, views the human psyche as being made up of several "parts" or "sub-personalities."

These inner parts may harbor contradictory impulses, feelings, or beliefs, which can cause internal conflict and emotional pain.

Parts Therapy is a technique used by hypnotists to help people connect with and comprehend their inner selves, which promotes harmony and resolution.

By addressing the various facets of who they are, people can strive for integration and lead more balanced and satisfying lives.

Children And Adolescent Hypnotherapy

Not only may hypnotherapy help adults, but it can also be quite helpful for kids and teenagers.

Because they may enter a hypnotic state naturally, children frequently respond well to hypnosis.

Younger clients receive hypnotherapy that is customized for their age and developmental stage.

It can help with problems like anxiety, phobias, incontinence, and behavioral disorders.

Hypnotherapists work with young clients to empower them with coping mechanisms, self-confidence, and emotional well-being in a way that is age- and child- appropriate.

Specialist hypnotherapy methods provide a wide range of tools to address emotional and psychological problems.

These methods demonstrate the versatility and therapeutic potential of hypnotherapy.

They include Age Regression, Past Life Regression, Parts Therapy, and Hypnotherapy for Children and Adolescents.

Even while some of these techniques might be regarded as strange or viewed with suspicion, they have proven to be beneficial in assisting people in discovering their inner selves, mending previous traumas, and achieving personal development.

CHAPTER SIX

Hypnotherapy's Ethical Considerations

Hypnotherapy Ethics

As a therapeutic technique, hypnosis has enormous potential to assist people in overcoming a variety of challenges, such as anxiety and phobias, weight control, and quitting smoking.

To protect clients' welfare and the integrity of the field, it must, like all forms of treatment, abide by a set of moral standards.

 Hypnotherapists must strictly adhere to many essential ethical principles, which are of utmost importance.

Educated Assent

Informed consent is one of the main ethical tenets of hypnotherapy. Therapists are required by law and morality to get their clients' express, informed consent before inducing hypnosis.

With this consent, consumers are guaranteed to be fully informed about the therapy's objectives, dangers, and procedures.

Moreover, it gives patients the freedom to decide for themselves whether or not to engage in hypnotherapy.

Since clients might not be aware of how much they are participating in therapy, a lack of informed consent might compromise their confidence in the therapist and result in ethical transgressions.

Protecting Privacy And Confidentiality

Another crucial ethical factor in hypnotherapy is protecting the privacy and confidentiality of clients.

Clients must experience a sense of security and certainty regarding the confidentiality of the personal information they divulge during sessions.

This confidentiality covers the client's hypnotherapy as well as the information discussed in the sessions.

The few situations in which private information may be revealed—such as when there's a chance the client or others could be harmed—are clearly outlined by ethical hypnotists.

During sessions, hypnotherapists must take precautions to guarantee their customers' security and privacy.

Promote transparency and trust between the therapist and the client, this entails setting up a cozy, quiet space that is unintimidated.

The efficacy and integrity of hypnotherapy depend heavily on ethical issues.

These factors include getting informed consent to guarantee clients' comprehension and autonomy during their therapeutic journey and upholding stringent privacy and confidentiality policies to protect clients' private information and mental health.

CHAPTER SEVEN

Self-Healing And Self-Management

Hypnotherapy has established a solid reputation as a legitimate therapeutic approach for treating a wide range of psychological and emotional issues.

Although professionally led traditional hypnotherapy sessions are beneficial, self-hypnosis has become more and more common as a self-care and self-improvement technique.

This essay will examine the idea of self-hypnosis and how it can be used to promote well-being and personal development.

Developing Auto-Hypnosis

The practice of putting oneself into a hypnotic state—a profoundly relaxed and highly suggestible state—is known as self-hypnosis.

Gaining confidence with self-hypnosis is a procedure that doesn't require a high level of psychology education.

There are numerous resources available that provide help in mastering this talent, such as books, online classes, and even apps for smartphones.

People usually learn to calm their bodies and thoughts through progressive muscle relaxation and deep breathing before beginning a self-hypnosis session.

When individuals reach a profound state of relaxation, they can use visualization methods or affirmations to help with anxiety, stress, or even pain relief.

People can become skilled at entering and staying in this trance-like state with practice.

Writing Scripts For Self-Hypnosis

Creating customized hypnosis scripts is a crucial component of self-hypnosis.

These scripts are intended to assist people in reaching their desired mental states and provide ideas for constructive change.

Writing a successful self-hypnosis script requires focus, accuracy, and knowledge of the problems that need to be resolved.

For example, if someone wants to get over their fear of public speaking, their script might offer tips for boosting confidence, lowering anxiety, and improving public speaking skills.

These scripts are created and refined using a highly customized process that enables people to customize their self-hypnosis sessions to meet their own needs.

Using Self-Improvement With Hypnosis

One powerful technique for improving oneself is self-hypnosis.

It can help people deal with stress, anxiety, and phobias, improve their self-esteem, and even deal with physical suffering by using pain management strategies.

It's an adaptable strategy that can be used to achieve a variety of individual objectives.

Self-hypnosis is a popular and affordable self-care technique that empowers people to take charge of their mental and emotional health.

But it's imperative to approach self-hypnosis methodically and patiently.

The greatest gains come from practice, just like with any other talent.

One useful tool for self-improvement and self-care is self-hypnosis.

Through the acquisition of self-hypnosis skills, the creation of customized scripts, and regular practice, people can realize their potential and bring about good transformations in their lives.

As they get more adept at using their minds, self-hypnosis turns into a useful tool for improving general well-being and personal development.

Research Studies On Hypnosis

Over the past few decades, hypnotherapy has been the subject of increasing scientific investigation, which has provided light on its efficacy and possible uses.

This growing corpus of research has shed important light on hypnosis's therapeutic advantages.

Hypnotherapy is a method that is based on actual research and is not just magical or pseudoscientific.

Its application for a variety of illnesses, including chronic pain, anxiety, quitting smoking, and managing weight, has been the subject of numerous research.

To explore the underlying mechanisms of hypnotherapy, these investigations use rigorous procedures such as neuroimaging techniques and randomized controlled trials.

Hypnosis as a supplement to conventional medical care is one area of great attention. Reducing reliance on medications and improving patient outcomes are two potential benefits of this integration.

For example, hypnosis has been investigated as a potential treatment for cancer side symptoms like pain and nausea. Studies have also looked into how it can improve surgical outcomes, such as less bleeding and faster recovery.

The neurological correlates of hypnosis have been the subject of a recent neuroscientific study, which has shed light on how the hypnotic state modifies brain activity.

Electroencephalography (EEG) and functional magnetic resonance imaging (fMRI) have revealed alterations in neural connections and the activation of particular brain regions during hypnotic sessions.

These results advance our knowledge of the brain processes behind hypnotherapy.

CHAPTER EIGHT

Hypnotherapy's Future

Since hypnosis is still developing and finding new uses, it seems to have a bright and varied future.

For the field, a few prominent directions and opportunities stand out:

Personalized Hypnotherapy: By better understanding the cognitive and psychological characteristics of each person, hypnotherapy can be tailored to meet their specific needs. More exact hypnotic inductions and recommendations are used in this.

Digital Hypnotherapy: The use of technology to improve the efficacy and delivery of hypnotherapy, including virtual reality and biofeedback.

These developments may increase the accessibility and personalization of therapy.

Neurofeedback and Hypnosis: This approach combines neurofeedback with hypnosis to give the client and therapist access to real-time data regarding brain activity.

Better outcomes and more focused interventions may arise from this combination.

Pain Management: More research on the use of hypnosis in pain relief, particularly about palliative care, chronic pain, and recovery after surgery.

Mental Health: Increasing the application of hypnotherapy to alleviate mental health issues like PTSD, depression, and anxiety disorders. combining hypnosis with established psychotherapy techniques to provide more thorough care.

Ethical Considerations: Further investigation is needed on the consent, possible hazards, and appropriate use of suggestive tactics in hypnotherapy, among other ethical elements of the practice.

Cross-Disciplinary Collaboration: Working together, hypnotists and medical specialists from different specialties create all-encompassing treatment regimens that use hypnosis as a supplemental modality.

Hypnotherapy's future will be determined by its incorporation into traditional medicine, which will be guided by cutting-edge methods and scientific study.

Hypnotherapy's potential as a therapeutic tool is expected to grow and diversify as our understanding of the mind and the brain deepens, opening up new pathways to better health and overall well-being.

Hypnotherapy: Unlocking The Subconscious Mind's Potential

Over the years, hypnotherapy—a distinctive and fascinating kind of therapeutic intervention—has become increasingly well-known and well-liked.

It entails assisting people in entering hypnosis, a deeply relaxing and focused state of awareness.

This treatment method makes use of the subconscious mind's capacity to treat a range of emotional and psychological problems. Although hypnosis is frequently portrayed in popular culture as a magical or mind-controlling technique, it is a well-researched, secure method that, when used by a qualified and moral practitioner, may produce noticeable results.

Comprehending The Hypnosis

The main component of hypnotherapy, hypnosis, is not something you see in Hollywood productions.

It's not about having people forget their names or cluck like chickens.

Instead, it is a highly suggestible and deeply relaxed state. While under hypnosis, people's attention is turned inward, but they nevertheless maintain complete awareness and control over their activities.

It's a state where the subconscious mind becomes more open to constructive suggestions and the critical, analytical mind recedes.

The Function Of The Subconscious Mind

Our subconscious is similar to the unseen force behind our feelings, ideas, and actions.

It holds memories, convictions, and feelings that frequently function below the surface, affecting our deliberate decisions and deeds. By utilizing the subconscious mind's ability, hypnotherapy enables patients to investigate and treat the underlying reasons for their issues.

Contexts For Hypnotherapy

There are numerous uses for hypnotherapy. It is frequently used to treat problems like anxiety, phobias, quitting smoking, losing weight, and even managing chronic pain.

Hypnotherapy can assist people in redefining problematic thinking patterns, overcoming limiting beliefs, and developing healthy behaviors by gaining access to the subconscious mind.

In the hands of qualified therapists, it can be a useful instrument.

The Healing Method

Generally, hypnotherapy is conducted in phases. The therapist evaluates the client's needs and goals during the first consultation.

The next step is the induction phase, where the client is led into a deeply relaxed condition.

When the client is in this state, the therapist can speak with their subconscious and provide constructive criticism and insights.

A debriefing and discussion of the experience round out the program.

Research And Effectiveness

The way hypnotherapy is portrayed in the media may make some people wary of it, yet research backs up its effectiveness in several settings.

Research has indicated that it can be especially helpful in reducing stress, managing pain, and easing anxiety.

Hypnotherapy's efficacy is frequently linked to its capacity to address the subconscious causes of psychological and emotional problems.

Conclusion

A distinctive and effective method for treating a variety of psychological and emotional problems is hypnotherapy.

People can gain insight into their inner workings, reframe harmful thought patterns, and create positive changes in their lives by leveraging the state of hypnosis and the subconscious mind.

For the best outcomes, it is imperative to find a licensed and moral practitioner. When used properly, hypnosis may be a great instrument for healing and personal development, giving people the ability to reach the full potential of their minds.